Circumcision

The Benefits and Risks Considerations for Parents

Harmony Royce

DEDICATION

To my friends and family, whose constant encouragement and support motivate me every day. This piece is a tribute to the support and affection you have given me along the way. With the hope that it will be a useful tool on your journey of self-discovery and development, I also dedicate this book to everyone.

DISCLAIMER

This book's content is meant primarily for educational and informational reasons; it is not meant to be used as professional, legal, or medical advice. If readers have any specific queries or concerns, they are advised to speak with trained professionals. Any direct, indirect, or consequential losses resulting from the use of this information are not covered by the author or publisher.

The views and experiences of the author are reflected in this book's content, which may not be representative of those of other people or organizations. Although every attempt has been taken to guarantee the authenticity of the material provided, neither the publisher nor the author can guarantee that the content is reliable or complete.

CONTENTS

ACKNOWLEDGMENTS..1

CHAPTER 1...1

A Historical and Cultural Perspective on Circumcision...........1

   1.1 The Cultural Origins of Circumcision................................. 1

   1.2 Circumcision Medicalization...3

   1.3 Circumcision in the Contemporary Era: A Health and Ethical

   Discussion..6

CHAPTER 2..10

Circumcision's Possible Health Benefits.............................. 10

   2.1 Lower Chance of UTIs (Urinary Tract Infections)....................... 10

   2.2 Lower Chance of STIs (sexually transmitted infections)............... 12

   2.3 Cervical and Penile Cancer Prevention................................14

CHAPTER 3..17

Additional Circumcision Health Benefits..............................17

   3.1 Balanitis and Balanoposthitis Prevention........................... 17

   3.2 Defense Against Paraphimosis and Phimosis..........................19

   3.3 Better Personal Hygiene.. 21

CHAPTER 4..24

A More Detailed Examination of the Dangers of Circumcision...........24

   4.1 Pain Both During and Following the Operation......................... 24

   4.2 Bleeding and Infection Risk...26

   4.3 Penis Injuries..28

CHAPTER 5..31

Concerns and Long-Term Issues..**31**

5.1 Inflammation of the Meatus, or Meatitis................................ 31

5.2 Sensation Loss.. 33

5.3 Emotional and Psychological Effects.................................... 35

CHAPTER 6..**38**

Circumcision of Infants: Ethical Issues.................................**38**

6.1 Consent and Bodily Autonomy..38

6.2 Cultural and Religious Aspects..40

6.3 The Pediatrician's Function in Making Decisions................. 42

CHAPTER 7..**46**

Public Health and Circumcision... 46

7.1 Circumcision in Campaigns for Public Health...................... 46

7.2 Circumcision's Economical Value.. 48

7.3 Juxtaposing Individual Risks and Population Benefits...................50

CHAPTER 8..**53**

Circumcision from the Viewpoint of Global Health.............**53**

8.1 Worldwide Circumcision Practices.. 53

8.2 International Circumcision Guidelines................................... 55

8.3 Circumcision and Human Rights..58

CHAPTER 9..**62**

Circumcision Alternatives.. 62

9.1 Treatment of Foreskin Disorders Without Surgery................62

9.2 Sanitary Procedures to Lower the Risk of Infection.............. 65

9.3 Instruction in Safe Sexual Behavior...................................... 67

CHAPTER 10..**71**

Making the Choice: A Parental Guide.. **71**

10.1 Assessing the Advantages and Dangers...71

10.2 Speaking with Health Care Experts...74

10.3 Honoring Individual Values and Family Traditions.....................76

ABOUT THE AUTHOR...**80**

ACKNOWLEDGMENTS

With great appreciation, I would like to thank everyone who helped me finish this book.

I want to express my gratitude to my family and friends for their everlasting belief in my goal, support, and encouragement. Throughout this journey, your love and understanding have been crucial.

I am particularly appreciative of my mentors and coworkers, whose knowledge and experience have improved my comprehension of the topic. I was inspired to push myself and pursue excellence by your advice and support.

We are grateful to the experts and scholars whose work served as the basis for this book for their devotion to learning and to expanding our comprehension of significant topics.

Lastly, I would like to express my gratitude to my readers. I'm motivated to share my ideas and observations by your participation and curiosity. I hope you find this book to be a useful tool for your trip.

CHAPTER 1

A HISTORICAL AND CULTURAL PERSPECTIVE ON CIRCUMCISION

1.1 The Cultural Origins of Circumcision

With roots in numerous civilizations and religions dating back thousands of years, circumcision is a practice with a rich historical tapestry. From a straightforward deed, it has developed into a sophisticated religious and cultural ritual with deep significance.

Historic Origins:

Circumcision was done as early as 2400 BCE in ancient Egypt, according to the earliest records. Men who were circumcised are depicted in Egyptian hieroglyphics; the practice was probably connected to social mores and religious rites. The spiritual significance of circumcision was highlighted by the belief that it purified the body and was frequently associated with the worship of deities.

Judaism's Religious Significance:

Circumcision, also known as **Brit Milah,** is a basic Jewish rite of passage that is carried out on the eighth day following the birth of a male infant. It marks Jewish identity and faith by representing the covenant that God made with Abraham. Prayers and festivities are held in conjunction with the ritual, highlighting its significance for the community.

As per Islamic customs:

Like Judaism, Islam places a great deal of religious significance on circumcision. Although the practice is not specifically required by the Quran, Muslims generally follow it as a Sunnah (the Prophet Muhammad's custom). It is frequently linked to purity and cleanliness, signifying a strong religious dedication.

Cultural Rituals in Different Societies:

In numerous communities around the world, circumcision takes many different forms outside of Abrahamic religions. It represents power, bravery, and social standing and is a rite of passage into manhood in various African and Aboriginal cultures. These rituals, which strengthen social ties and cultural identity, frequently include feasting, dancing, and group gatherings.

Differences Among Cultures:

Circumcision is performed for a variety of reasons. For example, it is a customary practice among several indigenous tribes in the Americas and Australia that is said to help people connect with their spiritual and ancestral worlds. On the other hand, some cultures emphasize personal expression by viewing circumcision as a type of body alteration similar to tattoos or body piercings.

1.2 Circumcision Medicalization

Perceptions of circumcision, especially in Western contexts, changed along with societies. The process began to become more medicalized in the 19th and 20th centuries, when it was framed in terms of health.

Influential Victorians:

Circumcision became popular in English-speaking nations throughout the Victorian era as a way to encourage cleanliness and stave against illness. Medical experts promoted circumcision as a defense against a number of illnesses, such as infections, phimosis (a disorder in which the foreskin is difficult to retract), and syphilis. Newborn male circumcision was encouraged by the time's dominant ideas of morality and hygiene.

The Medical Community and Health Claims:

Circumcision became a widespread hospital procedure in the early 20th century, especially in the US. The operation was approved by the American Medical Association, which claimed that it had substantial health benefits. According to medical professionals, circumcision lowers the risk of a number of illnesses, including penile cancer, STIs, and urinary tract infections.

Medical necessity versus routine practice:

Although circumcision was widely accepted, questions about its medical necessity started to surface. Many of the purported health benefits were questioned as study progressed. Well-known medical associations, such as the American Academy of Pediatrics, released recommendations indicating that although circumcision might have certain health benefits, it is not necessary for all males and should ultimately be left up to the parental choice.

Implications for Culture and Psychology:

Psychological factors were also introduced by the medicalization of circumcision. Studies have looked at the emotional effects of circumcision later in life, emphasizing emotions of physical autonomy being violated or lost. Since many people support a more customized approach to healthcare that respects individual choice, these conversations have led to a re-evaluation of the technique within the field of medical ethics.

1.3 Circumcision in the Contemporary Era: A Health and Ethical Discussion

Circumcision is still a controversial topic in today's society, with discussions mostly focused on individual rights, ethics, and health. The conversation is complex, encompassing a variety of ethical, medical, and cultural viewpoints.

The promotion of circumcision:

Circumcision proponents frequently highlight the health advantages of circumcision, pointing out that it may lower the risk of contracting specific infections and illnesses. They contend that the practice encourages good hygiene, especially in areas where there may be limited access to sanitary facilities and clean water. Furthermore, others argue that circumcision is a culturally appropriate decision that might improve sexual satisfaction for both partners.

Ethical and Opposition Issues:

On the other hand, opponents argue against regular circumcision, highlighting the significance of individual rights and bodily autonomy. Critics argue that there are serious ethical issues with doing surgery on a baby who is incapable of giving consent. Instead of promoting circumcision as a general policy, they favor informed parental choice, contending that parents should weigh the advantages and disadvantages of the procedure before making a decision.

The Function of Awareness and Education:

Educational programs that seek to give parents thorough information regarding circumcision have surfaced in recent years. These initiatives emphasize the importance of making well-informed decisions and urge parents to consider personal, cultural, and health-related aspects. These programs seek to enable families to make decisions that are consistent with their values and beliefs by encouraging candid conversations.

International Views and Methods:

Circumcision is a topic that is debated worldwide, not only in Western societies. Circumcision is a long-standing custom that is entwined with identity and belief systems in many cultures. The topic of how traditional traditions adjust to contemporary values and medical knowledge is being more and more discussed as globalization continues to impact cross-cultural interactions.

Directions for the Future:

Future conversations might center on developing more courteous and inclusive methods as society struggles with the effects of circumcision. A more complex view of circumcision in the contemporary world can be achieved by having discussions that respect various cultural customs while putting individual rights first.

Circumcision is a complex process with rich cultural, historical, and ethical facets that go beyond simple medical procedures. It is crucial that we approach the topic with tact, respect, and an appreciation for the various viewpoints that influence how we interpret this long-standing custom as we negotiate its intricacies.

CHAPTER 2

Circumcision's Possible Health Benefits

2.1 Lower Chance of UTIs (Urinary Tract Infections)

Because of anatomical variations, urinary tract infections (UTIs) are among the most prevalent infections among infants and early children, especially in females. However, studies show that male circumcised children are much less likely than their uncircumcised counterparts to get UTIs, particularly during the first year of life.

Research indicates that newborn boys who undergo circumcision have a tenfold lower risk of developing urinary tract infections compared to those who do not. Given that UTIs in men are very uncommon approximately 1% of male babies have one this finding is especially startling. There is a direct correlation between circumcision and urinary health, as seen by the lower prevalence of UTIs in circumcised infants.

The protection mechanisms are as follows:

There are a number of factors that contribute to this lower risk:

1. **These are some anatomical considerations:** An environment that is favorable to infections can be created by the foreskin's ability to retain moisture and bacteria. By removing this skin fold, circumcision lowers the risk of infection and bacterial colonization.

2. **Hygiene Advantages:** Because circumcision streamlines hygiene techniques, it is easier for caretakers to maintain cleanliness, especially for infants who are still learning to control their body functions. Proper hygiene can reduce the risk of UTIs in uncircumcised boys.

Clinical Consequences:

In some situations, especially when there is a family history of recurrent UTIs, some pediatricians and urologists recommend circumcision due to the possibility of fewer UTIs. The findings connecting circumcision to a decreased risk of this frequent infection, especially in early children, may reassure parents thinking about the operation.

2.2 Lower Chance of STIs (sexually transmitted infections)

Numerous studies have examined the connection between circumcision and the risk of STIs, and important results have indicated that circumcision may offer preventive advantages.

The following are the main findings:

Numerous studies in different populations, especially in Africa, have demonstrated that circumcision dramatically lowers the chance of contracting herpes simplex virus (HSV), HIV, and human papillomavirus (HPV):

1. **HIV:** According to research, men who are circumcised have a about 60% lower risk of acquiring HIV through heterosexual sexual activity than men who are not. This is explained by the removal of the foreskin, which has a high concentration of the virus's target cells and is hence more prone to infection.

2. **HPV:** Lower incidences of HPV infection, a major

contributor to cervical cancer in women, have also been linked to circumcision. Circumcision indirectly improves female partners' general health by lowering the risk of HPV transmission.

3. **HSV:** Research has shown that circumcised men had a lower prevalence of HSV, which adds credence to the idea that circumcision helps prevent STIs.

The following are some of the strategies that circumcision uses to prevent STIs:

1. **Elimination of the Foreskin:** The moist environment that the foreskin offers can help viruses survive and spread. By removing this favorable environment, its elimination lowers the likelihood of infection.

2. **Enhanced Hygiene:** Circumcision makes personal hygiene easier, lowering the amount of bacteria and viruses and making it simpler to wipe the penis. This is especially crucial in areas with potentially limited access to clean water.

3. **Reduction of Micro-abrasions:** Circumcision may lessen the number of micro-abrasions that occur during sexual activity, which might act as disease

entrance points.

Public Health Consequences:

Public health experts have highlighted the potential advantages of circumcision as part of larger measures to prevent STIs, particularly in areas with high infection rates, given the strong evidence linking it to lower STI rates. Nonetheless, the choice to get circumcised should always be discussed with medical experts while taking cultural norms and unique situations into consideration.

2.3 Cervical and Penile Cancer Prevention

A lower risk of some cancers, particularly cervical cancer in female partners and penile cancer in male partners, has been linked to circumcision. Despite the relative rarity of these diseases, it is important to consider the consequences of circumcision in preventing cancer.

Cancer of the Penile Region:

Poor hygiene, HPV infection, and phimosis, a condition in which the foreskin cannot be retracted are risk factors for penile cancer, a rare but dangerous cancer. According to research, men who have had circumcision are less likely to get penile cancer. This could be because of:

1. **Decreased HPV Exposure:** Circumcision may lower the risk of HPV-related penile cancer because it lessens the chance of HPV transmission.

2. Better hygienic practices are made possible by circumcision, which can further lower the incidence of infections and inflammation linked to penile cancer.

Female Partners' Cervical Cancer:

The main cause of the correlation between circumcision and the risk of cervical cancer is HPV transmission. Women who have circumcised partners are less likely to get HPV, which lowers their risk of cervical cancer. There are other ways to understand this relationship:

1. **Reduced Rates of HPV Transmission:** A decrease in the prevalence of high-risk HPV strains, which cause the majority of cervical cancer cases, has been associated with circumcision.

2. Male circumcised individuals may be more inclined to practice safer sexual behavior, which further lowers the risk of HPV transmission to female

partners.

Clinical and Research Suggestions:

Although there is strong evidence linking circumcision to a lower risk of cancer, it is crucial to remember that circumcision does not provide cancer prevention. Cancer prevention strategies continue to depend heavily on routine screenings, immunizations (such the HPV vaccine), and healthy lifestyle choices. In a larger framework of health and wellness, medical professionals may talk about circumcision as one of several aspects.

There are a number of possible health advantages of circumcision, including a lower chance of developing sexually transmitted diseases, a lower risk of urinary tract infections, and a lower chance of developing some types of cancer. To ensure that families can make well-informed decisions on the practice of circumcision, these advantages should be balanced against unique situations, cultural norms, and ethical issues.

CHAPTER 3

ADDITIONAL CIRCUMCISION HEALTH BENEFITS

3.1 Balanitis and Balanoposthitis Prevention

The glans, or head of the penis, and the foreskin are affected by the inflammatory diseases balanitis and balanoposthitis. Males who are not circumcised are more likely to suffer from these problems, mostly because they find it difficult to maintain good cleanliness.

Knowing the Difference Between Balanitis and Balanoposthitis:

1. **Balanitis** is the term for inflammation of the glans, which can be caused by a number of things, such as bacterial, viral, or fungal infections, irritants (such soaps or lotions), and underlying skin diseases (like psoriasis or eczema).

2. Inflammation of the glans and foreskin, frequently from similar causes, results in **Balanoposthitis**.

Redness, swelling, discharge, pain when urinating, and discomfort during sexual activity are some possible symptoms.

Circumcision as a Preventive Measure:

- By eliminating the foreskin, which can retain moisture and bacteria, circumcision can dramatically lower the likelihood of getting balanitis and balanoposthitis. This lessens the possibility of infections, which can cause inflammation.

- Male circumcised individuals are less likely to suffer from these inflammatory diseases, according to studies. Circumcision reduces the chance of irritants building up and causing infections by removing the foreskin, which also makes hygiene easier.

The following are some hygiene considerations:

- Males who are not circumcised must practice good hygiene in order to avoid developing balanitis and balanoposthitis. To properly clean the area, this involves pulling the foreskin back while taking a bath. Some people, however, might find this technique difficult, which could raise their risk of inflammation.

- Circumcision promotes general genital health by simplifying hygiene and reducing the likelihood of irritant buildup and infection.

3.2 Defense Against Paraphimosis and Phimosis

Foreskin disorders like phimosis and paraphimosis can cause severe discomfort and problems if left untreated.

Phimosis and Paraphimosis Definition:

1. Phimosis is the inability of the foreskin to retract over the glans. This disorder is common in babies, but if it continues throughout puberty or age, it could cause issues. Pain, trouble urinating, and recurring infections are some of the symptoms.

2. A more severe condition known as **paraphimosis** occurs when the foreskin retracts and cannot be brought back to its initial position. This may result in a medical emergency by causing pain, edema, and decreased blood flow to the glans.

Circumcision as a Solution:

- By completely removing the foreskin, circumcision successfully removes the danger of both phimosis and paraphimosis. These disorders cannot arise without a foreskin, avoiding the discomfort and possible consequences that come with them.

- Circumcision may be advised as a preventative measure for people who already suffer from phimosis or paraphimosis. This surgery not only fixes the current problem but also stops it from happening again.

Long-Term Implications:

- Circumcision can lessen the need for expensive and upsetting medical interventions like dilatation operations or emergency care by preventing phimosis and paraphimosis.

- The fact that circumcision can offer long-term protection against these potentially uncomfortable conditions may reassure parents thinking about having their sons circumcised.

3.3 Better Personal Hygiene

Maintaining good genital cleanliness is essential for general health, especially in avoiding infections and inflammatory diseases. Because the foreskin can retain germs and other infections, circumcision can improve hygiene practices.

Hygiene Issues in Males Who Are Not Circumcised:

- Males who have not been circumcised must practice certain hygiene habits to avoid infections, such as routinely pulling down the foreskin to completely clean the glans. Failing to do so may result in smegma accumulation, which is a mixture of dead skin cells and oils that can cause irritation and infections. Many people could find it difficult to regularly follow these hygiene guidelines, which could raise their risk of contracting diseases like balanitis or STDs.

Hygiene Benefits of Circumcision:

- Circumcision makes maintaining genital hygiene

easier. It is simpler to maintain cleanliness when the foreskin is absent since there is less room for smegma to grow.

- Due to better cleanliness habits made possible by the removal of the foreskin, studies show that circumcised guys typically report fewer genital irritation and urinary tract infections.

Cultural and Social Considerations:

- Circumcision is linked to cleanliness and sanitation in certain cultures, which reinforces social norms around genital care. Consequently, compared to their peers who are not circumcised, circumcised men might face fewer stigmas associated with genital cleanliness.

- The health benefits of circumcision can be further supported by educational programs that emphasize good hygiene habits. These programs can also encourage families to think about the procedure's possible benefits in terms of easier genital care.

Circumcision has other health advantages, such as better genital hygiene, protection from phimosis and paraphimosis, and the avoidance of balanitis and balanoposthitis. These advantages enhance the general health of male circumcision individuals, highlighting the significance of making an informed choice about the process. In order to make a decision that is consistent with their values and health concerns, families thinking about circumcision should examine these possible benefits in addition to their unique situation, cultural beliefs, and medical advice.

CHAPTER 4

A More Detailed Examination of the Dangers of Circumcision

4.1 Pain Both During and Following the Operation

Like any surgical intervention, circumcision is a medical operation that might cause some degree of pain and discomfort. For caretakers contemplating this treatment for infants or children, it is essential to comprehend the pain management procedures and the possibility of postoperative suffering.

The type of pain experienced during circumcision:

- To reduce any immediate pain, local anesthetic is usually used during the surgery. A number of methods can be employed, such as nerve blocks or topical anesthetics, which numb the area and lessen discomfort.

- Because they are unable to express their discomfort,

newborns may still experience some degree of distress during the surgical procedure even with anesthesia. To measure pain levels during the surgery, medical professionals frequently employ infant-appropriate pain scales, such as the Neonatal Infant Pain Scale (NIPS).

Postoperative Pain Management:

- As the local anesthetic wears off during circumcision, newborns may feel severe pain. According to studies, the first few days after surgery are crucial for pain management.

Strategies for managing pain that work well include:

1. **Analgesics:** Acetaminophen and other drugs can be administered to help reduce pain. Caregivers should heed the advice of medical professionals regarding the proper dosing.

2. **Comfort Measures:** Infants can be soothed during the recuperation period by skin-to-skin contact, gentle swaddling, or calming music.

3. **Observation:** Caretakers should be on the lookout for symptoms of extreme pain or discomfort, since they could point to issues that need medical

intervention.

The following are the long-term effects of pain:

- According to certain research, poor pain management during and after circumcision may result in heightened penile sensitivity and a later aversion to sexual engagement. Prioritizing efficient pain management techniques is crucial to reducing any potential long-term effects.

4.2 Bleeding and Infection Risk

There are hazards associated with every surgical treatment, and circumcision is no exception. It is essential to comprehend these dangers in order to make wise decisions.

Complications with Bleeding:

- Serious bleeding during circumcision is uncommon, but it might happen, especially if the procedure is carried out in a setting with insufficient surgical guidelines. Cutting into blood arteries or failing to sufficiently cauterize the surgical site might cause bleeding. The symptoms of excessive bleeding, such as persistent oozing or blood pooling in the diaper, should be communicated to parents and caregivers since they may require prompt medical intervention.

Risks of infection:

Another possible consequence linked to circumcision is infection. Although there is little chance of infection when the treatment is carried out by a qualified specialist in a sterile setting, things like inadequate hygiene or inappropriate aftercare can raise the risk.

Infection symptoms can include:

1. Swelling or redness surrounding the surgery site
2. Prolonged pain or discomfort
3. The release of pus or an unpleasant-smelling liquid
4. Lethargy or fever in the baby

Preventive Actions:

Caregivers should adhere to suggested aftercare protocols to reduce the risk of bleeding and infection. These protocols may include:

1. Maintaining a dry and clean environment
2. Regularly changing diapers to avoid moisture accumulation

3. Keeping an eye out for any indications of issues at the surgery site

Caregivers can better prepare for the procedure and react quickly to any potential complications by being aware of the risks of bleeding and infection.

4.3 Penis Injuries

When done by trained specialists, circumcision is usually safe, although in rare cases, difficulties may arise and the penis may sustain damage.

Types of Potential Injuries:

The patient's anatomy, the equipment utilized, or the surgical method can all lead to complications. Among the possible injuries are:

1. A tight circumcision is one consequence of excessive foreskin removal, which can cause discomfort and other health problems down the road.

2. **Incomplete Foreskin Removal:** Phimosis or the subsequent need for corrective surgery may result from insufficient foreskin removal.

Rarely, there may be unintentional damage to the surrounding tissues, which could result in scarring or difficulties that impair the penis's ability to function.

Implications of Injury:

Damage to the penis during circumcision may result in long-term consequences, including:

- Sexual activity-related pain or sensitivity
- Aberrant healing or scarring that may require additional medical attention
- Emotional or psychological effects associated with worries about the function or look of the genitalia

The significance of qualified practitioners is as follows:

Selecting a trained medical professional who has performed circumcision before is essential to lowering the chance of harm. Parents ought to also ask about the provider's training, background, and method of reducing difficulties.

- In addition to giving caregivers clarity on what to anticipate during and after the treatment, talking about potential hazards with the healthcare professional can help them be well-informed and ready.

Although circumcision may have a number of advantages, it is important to weigh the hazards involved, which include discomfort both during and after the surgery, the chance for infection and bleeding, and the potential for penile injury. In order to balance these dangers against the possible advantages and make an informed decision that is consistent with their interests and values, parents and caregivers should have candid conversations with medical specialists.

CHAPTER 5

CONCERNS AND LONG-TERM ISSUES

5.1 Inflammation of the Meatus, or Meatitis

Meatitis is an inflammatory disease that affects the meatus, which is the penis' entrance. Although circumcision is frequently done to reduce certain health risks, it can actually make this condition more likely to occur. It is crucial for those thinking about getting circumcised or for caregivers after the process to comprehend the mechanisms, symptoms, and available treatments.

Mechanism of Development:

- The foreskin's natural lubrication and protective layer are changed when it is removed. The glans, or head of the penis, is exposed in circumcised people, which may cause dryness and irritation. The risk of meatitis might be increased by poor cleaning and hygiene habits. This is especially important for newborns and young children, whose caretakers might not understand how important it is to keep the genital area clean.

The following are signs of meatitis:

- Redness and swelling at the meatus, pain or burning when urinating, and discomfort or irritation that may cause avoidance of urination, which could lead to more issues, are some possible symptoms.

- In extreme situations, meatitis may result in meatal stenosis, or scarring or narrowing of the meatus, which may necessitate surgery.

The following are common treatment options:

Management and Treatment:

1. **Improved Hygiene:** Frequent cleaning with mild soap and water can help prevent irritation.

2. Antibiotics or topical corticosteroids can be applied topically to treat infections and reduce inflammation.

3. **The use of medication:** Surgery to enlarge or repair the meatus may be required in chronic situations or where scarring develops.

4. In order to help circumcised guys avoid meatitis,

parents and other caregivers must be educated on good cleanliness habits.

5.2 Sensation Loss

One of the more contentious issues surrounding circumcision is the subject of penile sensitivity after the procedure. Although some research suggests a possible reduction in feeling, opinions differ widely, and the consequences can differ greatly from person to person.

Sensation and Nerve Endings:

- Sensitive nerve endings, especially Meissner's corpuscles, which are important for tactile perception, are highly concentrated in the foreskin. These nerve endings may be eliminated if the foreskin is removed, which could alter sensitivity. While some studies reveal no discernible difference between circumcised and uncircumcised males, others have claimed that circumcised men may be less sensitive during sexual activity.

Individual Variability:

Circumcision's effect on sensitivity might vary depending on a number of factors, such as:

1. **Age at Circumcision:** Compared to people who are circumcised in adolescence or adulthood, infants may experience distinct sensory consequences.

2. Subjective experiences can be influenced by psychological factors, such as expectations and perceptions about sensitivity.

3. **Healing Process:** Sensitivity levels may also be impacted by the body's post-circumcision healing and adaptation.

Less sensitivity may have an impact on one's ability to enjoy and be satisfied during sexual activity. While some men report experiencing less pleasure or having trouble achieving an orgasm, others indicate that their sexual experiences remain unchanged.

- Concerns about loss of sensitivity might be lessened by having candid conversations about sexual satisfaction and trying out other stimulation techniques.

5.3 Emotional and Psychological Effects

Circumcision has complicated psychological and emotional effects, which might be especially noticeable if the procedure is carried out against the patient's will during infancy. Feelings of regret, loss, or violation may result from the event, which may have an effect on a person's mental health and sense of self.

Views from a Cultural and Individual Perspective: Cultures and societies might have quite different views about circumcision. Circumcision may be considered unnecessary or even dangerous in some civilizations, while in others it is considered a vital health measure or a rite of passage.

- The lack of choice for those who were circumcised as infants can cause them to feel disconnected from their bodies as they age. Some people could have identity issues or be unsure of their masculinity.

Remorse Expression:

Men have been known to express regret for being circumcised, frequently expressing a sense of loss about their bodily autonomy. This may show up in a number of ways, such as:

- Anger-related feelings include frustration with parents or the medical establishment for denying them the option.

- A state of psychological distress Feelings of loss or violation can lead to problems like anxiety or despair.

- Online communities and support groups have grown in popularity as places for people to talk about their feelings and experiences while providing understanding and support to one another.

Importance of Counseling:

- Professional counseling or therapy can offer a secure environment for individuals grappling with the psychological effects of circumcision to examine their emotions and create coping mechanisms.

- In order to help people develop a healthy self-image and deal with any underlying problems resulting from the event, mental health specialists can help them navigate the emotions around circumcision.

It is important to take into account the possible long-term issues and problems, even though circumcision may be carried out for a variety of cultural and health-related reasons. People and families can make more educated decisions about circumcision if they are aware of issues like meatitis, the potential for diminished sensitivity, and the psychological effects of the procedure. In order to address these problems and make sure that people can deal with their experiences in a compassionate and understanding manner, open communication and support are essential.

CHAPTER 6

CIRCUMCISION OF INFANTS: ETHICAL ISSUES

6.1 Consent and Bodily Autonomy

The ethical discussion regarding neonatal circumcision revolves around the question of physical autonomy. According to the core idea of bodily autonomy, people should be free to make choices regarding their own bodies without outside pressure or interference. Because babies are unable to give informed permission, this principle becomes especially complicated when it comes to neonatal circumcision.

Informed Consent:

- In order to provide their voluntary consent, people must be able to comprehend the consequences of a medical operation. However, infants are unable to express their preferences or understand the ramifications of circumcision, therefore their parents or guardians must make the decision for them.

- Parents must make a decision that will affect their child for the rest of their lives. This calls into question whether it is morally acceptable to make decisions like this for someone else, particularly when that person is unable to express their views.

Philosophical Views:

Diverse philosophical systems offer differing viewpoints regarding consent in the circumcision of infants:

- The concept of deontological ethics This viewpoint emphasizes the ethics of deeds themselves. According to this perspective, it is always wrong to violate a child's physical autonomy, regardless of the cultural or medical rationale.

- The concept of consequentialism According to this ethical paradigm, an action's morality is determined by its results. Despite the lack of consent, proponents may contend that the operation is justified due to the possible health benefits of circumcision.

- **Care Ethics:** This method places a strong emphasis on connections and responsibilities, arguing that parents should behave in their children's best interests while also taking into account their eventual independence and preferences.

The Parental Responsibilities Role:

- Parents frequently feel pressured to make choices because of expectations from their families, cultures, or religions. Parents are urged by ethical considerations to critically assess these demands in light of the concepts of informed consent and bodily autonomy.

- A deeper comprehension of parental responsibility and the necessity of giving the child's future autonomy first priority can be facilitated by conversations about the long-term effects of circumcision.

6.2 Cultural and Religious Aspects

Circumcision has a strong religious and cultural foundation in many civilizations. These elements can make the ethical situation more difficult and have a big impact on how society views the surgery.

The Religious Importance:

- Circumcision, which represents a bond with God, is an essential religious rite for many Muslim and Jewish communities. The practice, called as **Brit Milah** in Judaism, is considered a commandment and is carried out on the eighth day of life. Islam views circumcision, or **Khitan**, as a Sunnah (advised practice) that denotes chastity and adherence to divine precepts. In many settings, circumcision is a religious practice with deep cultural and spiritual significance rather than just a medical operation. Healthcare professionals face an ethical dilemma in upholding these beliefs since they have to balance cultural sensitivity with medical ethics.

The following are examples of cultural norms and practices:

Circumcision is regarded as a sign of masculinity or a rite of passage in many cultures. For example, circumcision, which represents a boy's journey into manhood, is a feature of traditional initiation ceremonies among some African tribes. Parents' decisions can be greatly influenced by these cultural standards, which may cause some to put tradition ahead of scientific data. Healthcare professionals must promote educated decision-making while acknowledging the significance of these cultural beliefs.

Ethical Considerations in Balance:

The moral conundrum is striking a balance between worries about needless medical procedures and respect for cultural customs. Advocates contend that without discounting their cultural customs, families should be informed about the possible hazards and advantages of circumcision. Healthcare providers can acknowledge the cultural significance of circumcision while facilitating candid conversations with families and giving them thorough information. By encouraging respect and understanding, this method empowers parents to make better decisions that take ethical and cultural values into account.

6.3 The Pediatrician's Function in Making Decisions

When it comes to helping parents navigate the difficult decision-making process surrounding baby circumcision, pediatricians are essential. Their participation is essential to guaranteeing that families have the knowledge they need to make wise decisions.

It is the responsibility of pediatricians to provide concise, fact-based information regarding circumcision, including its possible advantages, disadvantages, and available options. This comprises:

- The potential medical benefits, including decreased risks of STIs and urinary tract infections, are discussed.

- **Risks and Complications:** describing potential immediate and long-term issues, such as discomfort, bleeding, and psychological impacts.

- **Cultural and Religious Contexts:** Addressing medical issues while acknowledging the cultural and religious significance of circumcision.

Respecting Family Values:

- When talking about circumcision, pediatricians must respect families' values and beliefs. Active listening, empathy, and knowledge of the family's cultural history and personal beliefs are all necessary for this.

- Pediatricians can develop trust with families by promoting open communication, which allows them to talk about delicate subjects without fear of criticism.

Managing Parental Pressure:

- When making a decision on circumcision, parents may encounter pressure from relatives or cultural norms. By offering a secure environment where parents may voice their worries and wishes, pediatricians can assist parents in navigating these demands.
- Providing assistance in making choices that are consistent with their values and the child's best interests.

Encouraging parents to participate in a shared decision-making process gives them the ability to actively participate in their child's medical care. Pediatricians can help with this process by:

- Encouraging parents to consider the benefits and drawbacks of circumcision in light of their particular situation.

- Emphasizing how crucial it is to take the child's future autonomy into account while making medical decisions.

There are many different ethical difficulties regarding infant circumcision, including intricate questions of physical autonomy, cultural significance, and healthcare workers' obligations. Pediatricians can assist families in making decisions that respect cultural values and medical evidence by skillfully and sensitively negotiating these moral conundrums. Infant circumcision is a topic of continuous discussion, which is necessary to guarantee moral behavior that puts children's welfare and autonomy first.

CHAPTER 7

PUBLIC HEALTH AND CIRCUMCISION

7.1 Circumcision in Campaigns for Public Health

In a number of places, including sub-Saharan Africa, where it is advocated as a means of preventing the spread of HIV and other STIs, circumcision has been incorporated into public health campaigns. Research showing that male circumcision can lower the risk of HIV acquisition among heterosexual men lends credence to the reasoning behind these efforts.

HIV Prevention Strategy:

Circumcision has been shown in numerous studies, including randomized controlled trials, to lower the risk of HIV infection in heterosexual men by about 60%. The removal of the foreskin, which is more prone to microtears during sexual activity, is thought to be the cause of this notable reduction in viral entry risk. Circumcision is seen as an essential part of a comprehensive prevention plan that includes condom use, education, and routine testing in areas with high HIV prevalence.

Circumcision programs targeting adult males and adolescents have been established in countries including South Africa, Kenya, and Uganda. These programs are frequently complemented by teaching on HIV awareness and safe sexual behaviors.

Typical campaign components include:

1. Community mobilization to promote involvement.

2. To improve accessibility, free or heavily discounted circumcision services are being offered.

3. Involving influential people and local leaders to promote the process in local communities.

Ethical Considerations:

- Although circumcision clearly improves public health, there are moral conundrums pertaining to individual rights. Campaigns for public health must guarantee that people are fully aware of the procedure's consequences and that participation is entirely voluntary.

- People must be made aware of the advantages and possible risks of circumcision in order for them to provide their informed consent. Transparency and respect for individual autonomy in decision-making should be the goals of campaigns.

7.2 Circumcision's Economical Value

A significant factor to take into account is how cost-effective circumcision is, particularly in areas with limited health resources. The long-term advantages of circumcision must be weighed against the procedure's initial expenses when analyzing its economics.

Economic Evaluation:

- Circumcision can be a financially advantageous intervention in areas with high HIV and STI incidence. For example, a South African study discovered that the cost of circumcision to prevent HIV infection is substantially less than the lifetime expenditures of HIV treatment.
- The direct expenses of the circumcision operation (surgical costs, facility fees, post-operative care) are

frequently taken into account in cost-effectiveness evaluations.

- The possible financial benefits of lowering the prevalence of HIV and STIs, which over time may result in cheaper medical expenses.

The effect on public health systems is as follows: Circumcision can lessen the strain on healthcare systems by lowering the prevalence of HIV and STIs, freeing up resources for other important health concerns. In environments with limited healthcare resources, this can be very advantageous.

Low-Risk Populations:

- The cost-benefit analysis for routine circumcision might not be as good in populations with low incidence of STIs and HIV. In these situations, the prevalence of diseases like penile cancer is usually minimal, which lessens the justification for the widespread use of circumcision.
- Instead of promoting circumcision as a panacea, public health programs should concentrate on focused interventions, stressing education and

preventive measures that correspond with the unique health requirements of the community.

7.3 Juxtaposing Individual Risks and Population Benefits

Although circumcision can have a lot to offer the public's health, these benefits must be weighed against the procedure's possible hazards to individuals and ethical issues. To guarantee that circumcision stays a personal, informed, and voluntary decision, public health initiatives must negotiate this complicated terrain.

Evaluating Individual Risks:

- Circumcision-related consequences for an individual may include discomfort, bleeding, infection, and long-term issues like sensitivity loss. It is imperative that these concerns be openly communicated in public health initiatives.

- To ensure that people may make informed decisions about their health, informed consent procedures should involve thorough conversations about the possible short- and long-term risks.

Ethical Imperatives:

People should not be forced to get circumcised because of social pressures or false beliefs about its health benefits. This is a requirement of ethical public health practice. As a public health measure, campaigns should encourage educated decision-making rather than requiring circumcision. It is impossible to overestimate the significance of culturally sensitive methods. Messages that are adapted to communities' values and beliefs can promote an atmosphere that is conducive to making well-informed decisions.

- The preservation of individual rights in public health efforts requires the maintenance of a voluntary approach. Without forcing the surgery on people or families, campaigns should promote conversations regarding circumcision.
- Providing educational materials outlining the advantages and disadvantages of circumcision is one possible strategy.
- Providing support networks, such as access to counseling and medical treatment, for those who

decide to have the operation.

Circumcision has a complex role in public health that combines ethical and individual rights concerns with substantial health benefits. Public health campaigns can successfully promote circumcision as a health intervention while upholding people's autonomy and rights by encouraging voluntary involvement, cultural sensitivity, and informed permission. The continuous discussion about circumcision in public health must change to reflect the most recent scientific findings as well as the shifting demands of communities.

CIRCUMCISION FROM THE VIEWPOINT OF GLOBAL HEALTH

8.1 Worldwide Circumcision Practices

Religious convictions, cultural standards, and medical procedures all have an impact on circumcision traditions, which vary greatly among civilizations and geographical areas. Gaining knowledge of these worldwide customs helps one to comprehend the wider effects of circumcision on society and health.

Regional Differences:

North America:

- In the US, between 60 and 80 percent of male neonates are circumcised, making it a rather prevalent practice. Cultural traditions and purported health benefits, like a lower risk of STIs and urinary tract infections (UTIs), are frequently associated with the practice. Circumcision rates, on the other hand, have been falling due to shifting perceptions of the practice and heightened understanding of the need for informed consent.

The European continent: Circumcision is less common in most European nations and is usually carried out for religious purposes, mostly by Muslim and Jewish groups. The overall prevalence is far lower than in the United States, which is frequently explained by cultural differences in beliefs about medical need and physical autonomy.

- Circumcision rates are especially low in the UK, where estimates place the number of circumcised boys at only 10% to 15%. Circumcision is not usually advised by the National Health Service (NHS), which believes that most boys do not need it.

North Africa and the Middle East:

- Circumcision is common in many of these nations, frequently as a religious rite of passage. Circumcision is typically carried out soon after birth or in early infancy and is considered by Muslims to be a Sunnah (a tradition of the Prophet Muhammad).

The practice in these areas is also supported by cultural views on moral upbringing and hygiene.

In many African communities, circumcision is common as a religious rite and a rite of passage into manhood. This is especially true in Sub-Saharan Africa. It is essential to social identity and belonging in some groups.

- Male circumcision is promoted by public health campaigns in a number of African countries as a way to prevent HIV transmission, in line with cultural customs that support health advantages.

Emerging Practices:

- In many societies, debates concerning the propriety of non-consensual newborn circumcision have been sparked by growing knowledge of human rights and ethical issues. Movements supporting informed consent and patient autonomy over medical procedures have resulted from this.

8.2 International Circumcision Guidelines

Cultural views, medical evidence, and public health

policies all have an impact on the medical community's approach to circumcision, which differs greatly between nations. Health professionals and legislators can learn about best practices by being aware of these principles.

The United States:

Supportive Guidelines:

- Circumcision is supported by groups such as the American Academy of Pediatrics (AAP), which states that although the health benefits are not strong enough to support universal circumcision, it might be advantageous for some groups, especially in regions with high HIV and STI rates.

- The significance of parental choice and informed permission is emphasized in the recommendations, which also acknowledge that parents should be informed about the dangers as well as the possible advantages.

The Royal Australian College of General Practitioners recognizes the potential advantages of routine circumcision in certain situations, especially for preventing infections or in families with a strong cultural or religious inclination towards the practice, but does not advise it for all males.

Warning Recommendations:

Europe and the United Kingdom:

- Routine circumcision for non-medical purposes is not advised by the National Institute for Health and Care Excellence (NICE), which instead aims to provide families with the necessary information so they can make an informed choice.

- With a heavy emphasis on the child's rights, several European standards take a cautious approach to circumcision, highlighting the need for informed consent and a good medical basis.

The World Health Organization, or WHO: The World Health Organization acknowledges the possible health advantages of circumcision in lowering the risk of STIs and HIV in areas with high prevalence. Nonetheless, it recommends that the operation be performed under the supervision of qualified medical personnel and in a clean, safe environment.

- According to WHO standards, community participation and education are essential to ensuring that people are aware of the consequences of circumcision and may make educated decisions regarding their health.

8.3 Circumcision and Human Rights

Important human rights issues are brought up by the practice of circumcision, especially in relation to children's rights and bodily autonomy. The consequences of circumcision are coming under more and more scrutiny as worldwide debates over ethics and human rights develop.

Proponents of bodily autonomy contend that non-consensual neonatal circumcision infringes upon people's fundamental freedom to make decisions regarding their own bodies. It is argued that infants are incapable of giving informed permission, which is a fundamental component of ethical medical practice.

- Children's rights movements emphasize how crucial it is to give people the freedom to choose whether or not to get circumcised when they are old enough to do so, giving them control over their bodies.

The rights to culture and religion: Critics of outright prohibitions on circumcision contend that for many cultures, it is an important religious and cultural ritual. It may be argued that attempts to restrict or control circumcision violate cultural liberties and rights.

- For legislators and healthcare professionals, finding a balance between upholding individual rights and honoring cultural customs is a difficult ethical dilemma.

A major global movement opposing non-consensual newborn circumcision is underway, with proponents urging legislative changes to safeguard children's rights. These movements place a strong emphasis on education, informed consent, and the necessity of a medical rationale for circumcision procedures on infants. Some nations have started looking into legislative frameworks to control the practice and make sure it is done in a way that respects children's rights while taking cultural and religious customs into account.

Views from a Global Perspective: The debate over human rights and circumcision is a subset of larger discussions concerning cultural sensitivity and medical ethics. Human rights activists and international health groups are realizing more and more how important it is to have thoughtful conversations that respect local customs while putting individual rights first.

- When considering circumcision procedures, the international community should take into account the United Nations Convention on the Rights of the Child, which highlights the importance of protecting children's rights, especially their right to bodily integrity.

Circumcision customs worldwide represent a nuanced interaction of religious, cultural, and medical factors. Regional views and the dominant medical culture have a significant impact on international guidelines. The discussion around circumcision is still shaped by the changing rhetoric on human rights and bodily autonomy, which calls for a delicate balancing act between preserving individual rights and honoring local customs. In order to promote educated decision-making in the best interests of people and public health, health professionals, legislators, and communities must traverse these issues with sensitivity and knowledge as worldwide attitudes on circumcision continue to change.

CHAPTER 9

CIRCUMCISION ALTERNATIVES

9.1 Treatment of Foreskin Disorders Without Surgery

For many years, phimosis (the inability to retract the foreskin) and balanitis (inflammation of the glans) have been treated surgically with circumcision. Nonetheless, there is increasing awareness of efficient non-surgical treatment alternatives that can treat these conditions and protect the foreskin.

Options for Non-Surgical Treatment

1. The mechanism of action of topical steroids is as follows: Topical steroids can help the foreskin loosen and minimize irritation. They reduce the swelling and discomfort brought on by phimosis and balanitis by inhibiting the local immunological response.

- **Application:** A topical steroid cream, like

hydrocortisone or betamethasone, is frequently prescribed by doctors to be administered directly to the afflicted area. For best results, this treatment is usually used in conjunction with mild stretching exercises.

- **Efficacy and Duration:** Studies have indicated that between 70 and 90 percent of patients respond favorably to a course of treatment, which typically lasts a few weeks and enables the foreskin to retract without the need for surgery.

2. Soft Stretching Activities:

- **Justification:** The foreskin can be made more elastic and retraction-friendly by gently stretching it. Children with phimosis benefit most from this approach.

- **The technique is as follows:** When the skin is more malleable after a warm bath or while bathing, parents or other caregivers can be taught to gently retract the foreskin. To prevent pain or harm, this procedure should be carried out gradually and without force.

- **Advice from Medical Professionals:** To make sure

the child is comfortable and that the practice is performed safely, healthcare professionals can provide advice on the frequency and method of stretching exercises.

3. Antibiotics for Balanitis:

- **Indications:** Antibiotics can successfully treat bacterial infections that cause balanitis without the need for circumcision. Depending on how serious the infection is, a doctor may prescribe oral or topical antibiotics.

- **Hygiene Education:** To prevent recurring infections, patients should also be educated on good hygiene habits. This may include advice on avoiding irritants and making sure the genital area is cleaned thoroughly.

4. Follow-Up Care:

- **Regular Monitoring:** To evaluate the efficacy of non-surgical treatments and guarantee that any consequences are promptly handled, follow-up with a healthcare professional is necessary on an ongoing basis.

- **Education of Patients:** It is important to teach patients and their families how to spot symptoms of treatment failure or consequences, such as ongoing pain, strange discharge, or changes in the foreskin's appearance.

9.2 Sanitary Procedures to Lower the Risk of Infection

For uncircumcised males, maintaining good genital cleanliness is essential to avoiding infections and irritation. Frequent cleaning procedures assist reduce the likelihood of problems that circumcision frequently attempts to prevent in addition to promoting general genital health.

The Value of Personal Hygiene

The first step is to comprehend the foreskin: If not adequately cleaned, the delicate foreskin can retain bacteria and debris. Urinary tract infections (UTIs) and balanitis are among the infections that are made more likely by this.

- Teaching caregivers the value of washing under the foreskin as part of daily hygiene routines is crucial.

2. Hygienic Practices:

Daily Cleaning:

- Promote washing the genital area with warm water every day while taking a bath. If at all feasible, parents of younger children should gently pull back the foreskin and clean underneath it to get rid of debris and smegma, a natural fluid.

- Use unscented, gentle soap to prevent irritation. Because they can make sensitivities worse, harsh soaps and irritants should be avoided.

During Childhood:

- As soon as the child feels at ease with the procedure, parents should start teaching them good hygiene habits. Emphasizing gentle handling is crucial to preventing discomfort or agony.

- As kids get older, teach them how to take care of themselves by emphasizing the value of keeping the space clean every day.

3. Avoidance of Infections:

- The risk of infections, such as UTIs and balanitis, can be considerably decreased by practicing good hygiene. Frequent cleaning helps stop bacteria and other pathogens from growing, which can cause illness and irritation.

- If necessary, early medical intervention can be prompted by education on how to identify infection symptoms including redness, swelling, or discharge.

4. Cultural Sensitivity:

- Health education ought to be culturally aware and customized to accommodate various groups' needs and values. Having conversations about hygiene with healthcare professionals and community leaders might encourage acceptance and adherence to advised measures.

9.3 Instruction in Safe Sexual Behavior

Circumcision is only one tactic among many used to prevent sexually transmitted infections (STIs). In order to lower the risk of STIs for both circumcised and uncircumcised males, it is critical to emphasize safe sexual behaviors, including the regular use of condoms.

Appropriate Sexual Behavior

1. Use of Condoms:

- **Efficacy:** The risk of STIs, including HIV, is considerably decreased by using condoms correctly and consistently. During sexual action, they operate as a physical barrier to stop direct contact and the exchange of bodily fluids.

- **Instruction on Usage:** Instructions on how to use condoms correctly, including how to check expiration dates, use them correctly, and dispose of them, should be part of comprehensive sex education programs.

2. Regular STI Testing:

- **Importance of Testing:** People who engage in sexual activity, particularly with several partners, should get screened for STIs on a regular basis. Better health outcomes can be achieved and the spread of infections can be stopped with early detection and treatment.

- **Access to Testing:** Public health programs should work to make STI testing more widely available and reasonably priced, particularly for high-risk groups. Testing in clinics, community centers, and schools is part of this.

3. Interaction with Partners:

- **Promoting Free Discussion:** Open communication regarding sexual health, including STI status and testing history, should be promoted between individuals and their partners. This promotes shared health habits and a sense of accountability.

- **Talking about Safe Practices:** More responsible sexual conduct and a lower risk of STIs can result from empowering people to talk about and negotiate safe sex practices.

Education and Awareness Campaigns:

- **Public Health Initiatives:** Regardless of a person's status as circumcised, comprehensive sexual education programs can play a significant role in educating them about the significance of safe sexual behaviors. Different age groups and ethnic backgrounds should be the focus of these programs.

- **Technology Utilization:** Online platforms and social

media can be useful instruments for raising awareness of STIs and spreading information about safe sexual practices.

5. Cultural Competence:

- **Personalized Methods:** Culturally responsive sexual health education should respect other groups' customs and beliefs while encouraging safe behaviors. Involving local authorities and medical specialists can improve the efficacy of educational initiatives.

Non-surgical therapy methods, good hygiene habits, and instruction on safe sexual practices offer good alternatives to circumcision, which is still a prevalent intervention for a number of medical issues. By highlighting these tactics, medical professionals may reduce risks and preserve the foreskin while empowering people and families to make educated decisions regarding their health. In order to guarantee that these alternatives are recognized, embraced, and successfully applied in communities, comprehensive education and public health programs are essential.

CHAPTER 10

MAKING THE CHOICE: A PARENTAL GUIDE

10.1 Assessing the Advantages and Dangers

Parents must thoroughly weigh the possible advantages and disadvantages of circumcising their child before making the decision. This is a complex decision with personal, ethical, and medical aspects.

Recognizing the Advantages

1. Medical Benefits:

- **Decreased Infection Risk**: It has been demonstrated that circumcision reduces the likelihood of UTIs in infancy, especially in boys who are predisposed to them due to anatomical problems. Research shows that compared to their counterparts who are not circumcised, circumcised newborns had a much lower incidence of UTIs.

- **Decreased Presence of Specific STIs:** Circumcision may lower the chance of contracting HIV and other sexually transmitted illnesses, according to some study. Removing the foreskin may reduce the risk of transmission during sexual activity because it is thought to offer a possible entrance site for viruses.

- **Prevention of Foreskin-Related Conditions:** Conditions like balanitis (inflammation of the glans) and phimosis (inability to retract the foreskin), which can cause discomfort and consequences requiring medical attention, can be avoided by circumcision.

2. Social and Cultural Aspects to Take Into Account: Circumcision is a deeply ingrained customary cultural or religious rite of passage for many households. It can be viewed as a way to strengthen identification and continuity with ancestors' customs while also fostering a sense of belonging to a specific group.

Recognizing the Dangers

1. Surgical Risks:

- Circumcision has inherent risks, such as bleeding, infection, and anesthesia-related problems, much like any other surgical treatment. Serious problems are uncommon, but they can happen and may necessitate further medical care.

- **Meatitis:** After circumcision, an inflammation of the meatus may develop, causing pain and discomfort when urinating.

2. Psychological and Emotional Considerations:

- Some people may feel regret or a sense of loss related to circumcision, especially if it was done during infancy without their consent. When making this choice for their child, parents must be aware of the possible emotional ramifications.

3. the loss of sensitivity: The possible decrease of penile sensation after circumcision is a topic of continuous discussion. According to several studies, the removal of the foreskin, which has delicate nerve endings, may result in less sensitivity when having intercourse later in life.

Considerations for Balancing

Parents need to carefully consider these advantages and disadvantages. Listing the benefits and drawbacks, talking about them with family members, and considering their values and views can all be beneficial. The decision will be well-informed and in line with the family's priorities thanks to this thoughtful process.

10.2 Speaking with Health Care Experts

Having conversations with medical experts is an essential part of the circumcision decision-making process. Urologists and pediatricians can offer insightful advice and guide parents through the challenges of this decision.

Looking for Expert Advice

1. thorough consultation: To talk about the particular medical, cultural, and ethical facets of circumcision, parents should make an appointment with a reputable pediatrician. Any queries or worries parents may have regarding the process can be discussed at this meeting.

- **Information Based on Evidence:** In order to assist

parents in making educated decisions, healthcare professionals can provide evidence-based information about the advantages and disadvantages of circumcision. They can also talk about other therapies for diseases like phimosis that can typically result in circumcision.

2. Comprehending Personal Situations:

- Since each child is different, decisions about circumcision should take into account each child's medical history. Any anatomical issues, such as congenital defects, that can affect the choice might be evaluated by pediatricians.

- It is important to urge parents to talk about their family history and any illnesses that might make circumcision necessary or cause them to have worries about the process.

3. Ethical Considerations:

- It is also essential to have a conversation regarding the ethical aspects of circumcision. The consequences of making a decision on behalf of a kid who is incapable of giving consent can be better understood by parents with the assistance of medical specialists.

- In order to help parents decide how best to reconcile cultural and personal values with medical guidelines, this discussion can also examine how these two areas cross.

10.3 Honoring Individual Values and Family Traditions

The choice to circumcise a child is often closely linked to family, religious, or cultural customs. Parents must respect these principles and incorporate them into their decision-making process.

Religious and Cultural Aspects

1. Knowing Traditions:

- Circumcision (Brit Milah) is a holy covenant and a fundamental part of Jewish faith for Jewish families. Parents can make better decisions if they are aware of the significance of this custom.
- A common and spiritually significant process in Islamic societies, circumcision (Khitan) is

sometimes seen as a rite of passage for young males.

2. Bringing Modern Medicine and Tradition into Balance:

- Parents should take into account contemporary medical viewpoints in addition to cultural and religious views, which are important. This calls for a careful balancing act, making sure that choices respect customs while taking into account the most recent research and health recommendations. Parents may consult community elders or religious leaders who are willing to talk about medical issues and can offer insight into the decision's cultural ramifications.

Individual Principles and Family Relationships

1. Talking About Values:

- Parents ought to be candid about their own personal views on circumcision. This entails investigating sentiments regarding medical ethics, cultural heritage, and bodily autonomy.

- Talking with family members can also assist resolve

conflicts and promote a cohesive approach to the choice.

2. Considering Future Implications:

- Parents should think about the potential emotional and physical effects of their choice on their child in the future. Talking about the child's potential feelings regarding their circumcision status when they get older may fall under this category.

- In order to ensure that their child knows the rationale behind their decision, parents must be ready to talk to them about it later in life.

3. Establishing a Helpful Environment: Whatever the option, it is important to create an environment that supports the child's identity and choices. In order to foster positive attitudes toward their child's physical self, parents should respect their sentiments and encourage candid discussions about their child's body.

In summary, the choice to get circumcised is intricate and multidimensional, involving thorough evaluation of personal, cultural, ethical, and medical considerations.

Parents are urged to consider the advantages and disadvantages, seek advice from medical experts, and honor the customs and values of their family. Parents can make an informed decision that supports their child's wellbeing and is consistent with their beliefs by approaching this decision carefully and cooperatively.

ABOUT THE AUTHOR

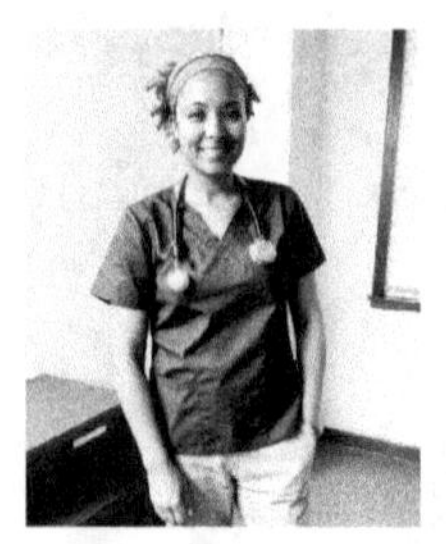 Harmony Royce is a dedicated healthcare worker who has a strong interest in holistic wellness. Harmony's extensive history in various aspects of health and wellness provides her with a wealth of knowledge and expertise that she can utilize in her writing and professional endeavors.

Harmony is a talented author who crafts thought-provoking books that inspire readers to have well-rounded, balanced lives. She writes about a variety of health-related topics, such as diet, exercise, mental health, and mindfulness. Her approachable writing style combines practical guidance with evidence-based research to make complex health concepts approachable and engaging for readers of all ages.

Harmony actively promotes the benefits of holistic health through writing, community workshops, and internet forums. Her mission is to educate and inspire people about the transformative power of self-care and healthy lifestyle choices.